LIVER

CIRRHOSIS

COOKBOOK

SARAH JACK

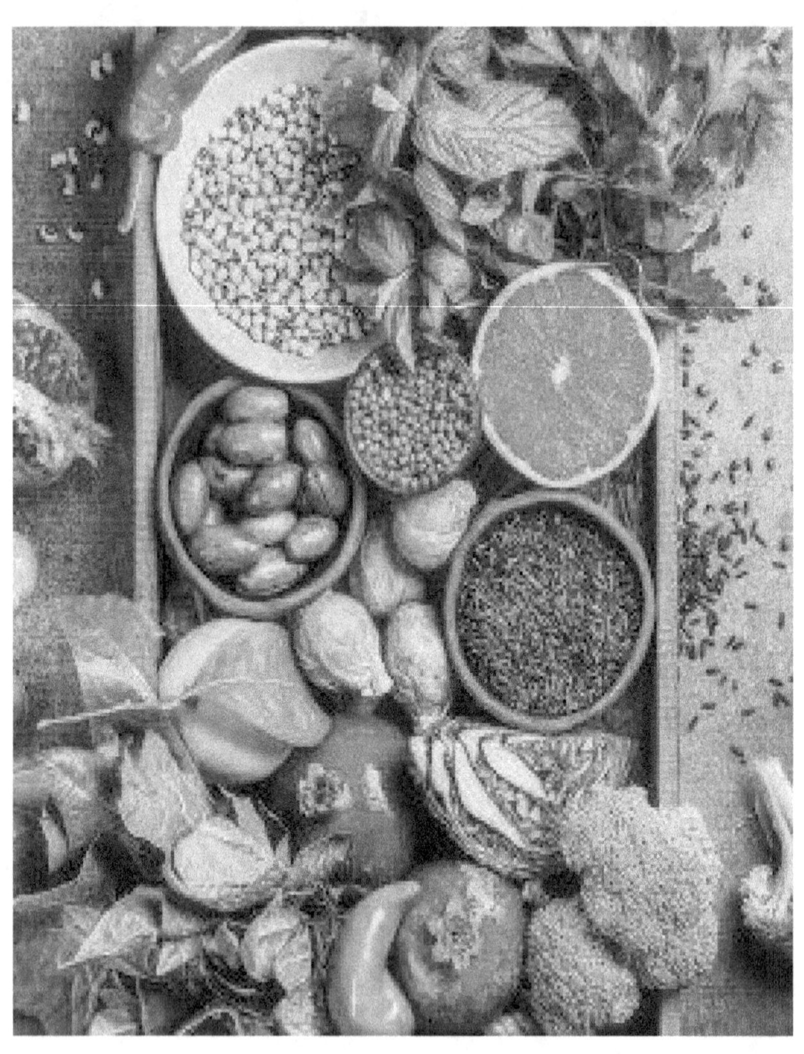

COPYRIGHT

All rights reserved. This book or any portion thereof may not be reproduced or used in any manner whatsoever without the express written permission of the publisher except for the use of brief quotations in a book review.

TABLE OF CONTENTS

INTRODUCTION

LIVER

The liver, positioned in the upper right abdomen below the diaphragm and above the stomach, is a pivotal organ fundamental for sustaining overall health and functionality. Here are several crucial aspects to grasp about the liver:

Metabolic Functions: The liver engages in a plethora of metabolic activities vital for generating energy and metabolizing nutrients. It regulates blood glucose levels by storing glucose as glycogen and releasing it as needed, and it governs lipid metabolism, encompassing the synthesis, breakdown, and transportation of fats and cholesterol.

Detoxification: A primary task of the liver involves detoxification, wherein it filters toxins, medications, alcohol, and metabolic byproducts from the bloodstream. These substances are metabolized and neutralized by the liver, converting them into less harmful compounds that are subsequently excreted through urine or bile.

Bile Production: Another critical function of the liver is bile production, a digestive fluid essential for fat digestion and absorption in the small intestine. Bile, stored in the gallbladder, is released during digestion to aid in fat emulsification, facilitating the absorption of fat-soluble vitamins and nutrients.

Protein Synthesis: The liver synthesizes proteins crucial for various bodily functions, including blood clotting factors, albumin for fluid balance regulation, and immune-related proteins. It also manufactures enzymes and hormones vital for metabolic processes and other physiological functions.

Nutrient Storage: Acting as a reservoir, the liver stores various nutrients such as glycogen (for glucose storage), vitamins like A, D, and B12, and minerals including iron and copper. These stored nutrients are released into the bloodstream as needed to maintain stable blood sugar levels and support overall metabolism.

Regeneration: Notably, the liver possesses remarkable regenerative abilities, capable of repairing and regenerating damaged tissue. Even after injury or partial removal, the liver can regenerate, reinstating its structure and function. This regenerative capacity is pivotal for recuperating from injuries, surgeries, or certain liver ailments.

Immune Function: Integral to the body's immune system, the liver filters and eliminates bacteria, viruses, and pathogens from the bloodstream. Additionally, it produces immune factors and proteins essential for combating infections and modulating immune responses.

Diseases and Disorders: A spectrum of diseases and disorders can impact liver health, ranging from acute conditions like hepatitis and liver infections to chronic ailments such as fatty liver disease, cirrhosis, and liver cancer. Factors contributing to liver disease encompass alcohol abuse, viral infections (e.g., hepatitis B and C), obesity, diabetes, and genetic predispositions.

In summary, the liver epitomizes a multifaceted organ undertaking critical roles in metabolism, detoxification, digestion, nutrient storage, and immune function. Upholding liver health through a balanced diet, regular physical activity, limited alcohol intake, and avoidance of harmful substances is paramount for overall well-being. Routine medical assessments and screening examinations play a pivotal role in early detection and management of liver diseases.

LIVER CIRRHOSIS

Liver cirrhosis is a chronic and progressive ailment marked by the formation of scar tissue within the liver, disrupting its normal architecture and function. Below is an outline of liver cirrhosis, encompassing its etiology, manifestations, complexities, diagnosis, and management:

Causes: Liver cirrhosis can stem from diverse origins, including chronic alcohol abuse, viral hepatitis (such as hepatitis B and C), non-alcoholic fatty liver disease (NAFLD), autoimmune liver disorders, hereditary conditions (like hemochromatosis and Wilson's disease), and prolonged exposure to toxins or specific medications.

Pathophysiology: Liver cirrhosis entails persistent liver injury triggering inflammation and the buildup of scar tissue (fibrosis) in the liver. As fibrosis advances, the liver becomes progressively nodular and hardened, impeding its normal function. This can result in complications such as portal hypertension, liver failure, and an elevated risk of liver cancer.

Symptoms: Liver cirrhosis may initially manifest without symptoms or with vague clinical signs. As the disease advances, common symptoms may encompass fatigue, weakness, abdominal discomfort, reduced appetite, nausea, weight loss, jaundice (yellowing of the skin and eyes), bruising or bleeding easily, leg or abdominal swelling (ascites), and cognitive impairment (hepatic encephalopathy).

Complications: Liver cirrhosis can precipitate several complications, including portal hypertension (elevated pressure in the portal vein system), culminating in varices (enlarged blood vessels) in the esophagus and stomach, heightening the risk of bleeding. Other complications entail ascites, hepatic encephalopathy (cognitive impairment due to toxin accumulation), liver cancer (hepatocellular carcinoma), and liver failure.

Diagnosis: Diagnosis typically integrates medical history, physical examination, liver function tests, coagulation studies, imaging modalities (ultrasound, CT scan, MRI), and occasionally liver biopsy to gauge the extent of liver damage and confirm the diagnosis.

Treatment: Treatment goals involve symptom alleviation, disease progression deceleration, and complication prevention. Essential lifestyle modifications encompass alcohol abstinence, adhering to a healthy diet, and avoiding substances harmful to the liver. Medications may be prescribed to manage specific symptoms or underlying causes, such as antivirals for hepatitis or immunosuppressants for autoimmune liver disorders. In advanced cases, liver transplantation may be imperative to replace the impaired liver with a healthy donor liver.

Prognosis: Prognosis hinges on the underlying cause, extent of liver damage, presence of complications, and treatment response. Timely diagnosis and intervention can ameliorate outcomes and enhance the quality of life for those with liver cirrhosis. Nevertheless, advanced cirrhosis may culminate in liver failure, necessitating transplantation or palliative care.

In essence, liver cirrhosis denotes a grave condition characterized by irreversible liver tissue scarring, leading to compromised liver function and potentially life-threatening complications. Timely identification, management of root causes, and appropriate medical intervention are pivotal for optimizing outcomes and enhancing the well-being of affected individuals.

LIVER CIRRHOSIS DIET

A liver cirrhosis diet customized to the needs of individuals with this condition is vital for symptom management, liver function support, and complication prevention. Here's a breakdown of dietary considerations for liver cirrhosis:

Moderate Protein Consumption: It's crucial to consume moderate amounts of high-quality protein like lean meats, poultry, fish, eggs, dairy, legumes, and tofu to aid in tissue repair and overall health. Distributing protein intake evenly throughout the day can ease the liver's workload.

Limit Sodium: Limiting sodium intake helps mitigate fluid retention and associated issues like ascites. Avoid processed foods, canned goods, salty snacks, and high-sodium condiments. Instead, flavor foods with herbs, spices, lemon juice, or vinegar.

Monitor Fluid Intake: Since fluid retention is common in liver cirrhosis, monitoring and potentially restricting fluid intake, especially in cases of swelling or ascites, is important. Seeking personalized recommendations from a healthcare provider is advisable.

Healthy Fats Inclusion: Opt for healthy fats such as those found in olive oil, avocados, nuts, and seeds, while limiting saturated and trans fats from processed and fried foods, as they can contribute to liver inflammation.

Increased Fiber Consumption: Including fiber-rich foods like fruits, vegetables, whole grains, legumes, and nuts supports digestion, regular bowel movements, and prevents constipation, but moderation may be necessary for those with advanced cirrhosis and complications like hepatic encephalopathy.

Alcohol Abstinence: Completely avoiding alcohol is essential to prevent further liver damage and the progression of cirrhosis.

Frequent Small Meals: Consuming smaller, more frequent meals throughout the day helps manage digestive discomfort, stabilize blood sugar levels, and provide a steady source of energy.

Vitamins and Minerals Supplementation: In cases where deficiencies exist due to impaired absorption or dietary restrictions, supplements like vitamin D, vitamin B12, or zinc may be recommended by healthcare providers.

Avoidance of Raw Seafood and Undercooked Meats: Individuals with liver cirrhosis are at a heightened risk of bacterial infections, making it important to steer clear of raw or undercooked seafood, meats, and eggs to prevent foodborne illnesses.

Collaborating closely with healthcare professionals, including a registered dietitian, is essential to establish and maintain a liver-friendly diet that meets nutritional requirements, supports liver function, and helps manage symptoms and complications associated with liver cirrhosis. Regular monitoring and adjustments to the diet may be necessary to optimize outcomes.

BENEFITS OF LIVER CIRRHOSIS DIET

The benefits of adhering to a liver cirrhosis diet tailored to meet the unique requirements of individuals battling with this ailment are numerous and significant. Below are some key benefits:

Supports Liver Function: A liver cirrhosis diet is formulated to alleviate the strain on the liver and bolster its performance. By furnishing essential nutrients in appropriate proportions, the diet aids in optimizing liver health and potentially decelerating the advancement of liver damage.

Manages Symptoms: Adjustments in diet can effectively handle symptoms commonly linked with liver cirrhosis, such as ascites, fatigue, nausea, and diminished appetite. Addressing these symptoms can lead to enhanced comfort and an overall sense of well-being.

Prevents Complications: Adhering to a liver cirrhosis diet diminishes the likelihood of complications associated with the condition, including hepatic encephalopathy, portal hypertension, and variceal bleeding. By fostering liver health and minimizing strain on the liver, the diet helps mitigate the risk of adverse outcomes.

Maintains Nutritional Status: Liver cirrhosis can disrupt the body's ability to absorb and utilize nutrients efficiently. A meticulously devised diet ensures individuals receive adequate nutrition despite potential hindrances in digestion and absorption, thus thwarting malnutrition and bolstering overall health.

Reduces Liver Inflammation: Certain dietary constituents, such as healthy fats and antioxidants sourced from fruits and vegetables, possess anti-inflammatory attributes that may alleviate liver inflammation linked with cirrhosis.

Incorporating these foods into the diet could lead to diminished inflammation and associated symptoms.

Promotes Digestive Health: A liver cirrhosis diet often encompasses high-fiber foods, which foster digestive health and regular bowel movements. Fiber aids in averting constipation, a prevalent issue among individuals with cirrhosis, and supports gastrointestinal function.

Enhances Quality of Life: By addressing nutritional needs, managing symptoms, and curbing the risk of complications, a liver cirrhosis diet significantly betters an individual's quality of life. Enhanced comfort, heightened energy levels, and an overall sense of well-being contribute to an improved quality of life despite contending with a chronic ailment.

Empowers Individuals: Adhering to a specialized diet empowers individuals with liver cirrhosis to actively participate in managing their health and well-being. By making informed dietary choices and adhering to dietary recommendations, individuals gain control over aspects of their condition and optimize their health outcomes.

A liver cirrhosis diet offers myriad benefits that advance liver health, symptom management, and overall quality of life for individuals navigating this condition. It serves as an integral facet of comprehensive management and treatment approaches for liver cirrhosis, supplementing medical interventions and lifestyle modifications.

EXERCISE AND LIVER HEALTH

Regular physical activity plays a pivotal role in enhancing liver health and overall wellness. Here's how exercise contributes to the well-being of the liver:

Weight Management: Engaging in regular physical activity aids in maintaining a healthy weight or achieving weight loss, which is vital for liver health. Excessive body weight, particularly visceral fat surrounding the abdomen, is closely linked to fatty liver disease and liver inflammation. By facilitating weight loss and reducing fat deposition in the liver, exercise helps prevent or manage fatty liver disease.

Enhances Insulin Sensitivity: Exercise improves insulin sensitivity and glucose metabolism, lowering the risk of insulin resistance and type 2 diabetes. Insulin resistance is a significant factor in non-alcoholic fatty liver disease (NAFLD) and can lead to liver inflammation and scarring. By boosting insulin sensitivity, exercise assists in preventing NAFLD and slowing down the progression of liver damage in individuals with existing liver conditions.

Reduces Liver Fat: Studies have demonstrated that aerobic exercise can decrease liver fat content in individuals with fatty liver disease. Engaging in regular aerobic activities such as brisk walking, jogging, cycling, or swimming enhances energy expenditure and facilitates the mobilization of stored fat, including fat accumulated in the liver. This leads to a reduction in liver fat levels and an improvement in liver function over time.

Promotes Detoxification: Exercise stimulates blood circulation and augments blood flow to the liver, aiding in the elimination of toxins and metabolic waste products from the body. Enhanced blood flow supports liver function and assists in its detoxification processes, facilitating the removal of harmful substances and promoting overall liver health.

Reduces Inflammation: Chronic inflammation is a hallmark of liver diseases like hepatitis, fatty liver disease, and liver cirrhosis. Regular exercise exerts anti-inflammatory effects, diminishing systemic inflammation and reducing levels of inflammatory markers in the body, including those associated with liver inflammation. By alleviating inflammation, exercise safeguards liver cells from damage and hinders the progression of liver diseases.

Enhances Immune Function: Exercise boosts immune function and fortifies the body's defense mechanisms against infections and diseases. A robust immune system plays a pivotal role in shielding the liver from pathogens, viruses, and other harmful agents that could induce liver damage. Regular exercise sustains immune function and bolsters liver health.

Improves Blood Lipid Profile: Exercise has the potential to enhance blood lipid profile by elevating levels of HDL (good) cholesterol and reducing levels of LDL (bad) cholesterol and triglycerides. Dyslipidemia is a prevalent risk factor for fatty liver disease and cardiovascular complications. By enhancing lipid metabolism, exercise curtails the accumulation of fat in the liver and diminishes the risk of liver-related and cardiovascular ailments.

Incorporating regular exercise into one's lifestyle is imperative for maintaining optimal liver health. Strive for at least 150 minutes of moderate-intensity aerobic exercise or 75 minutes of vigorous-intensity aerobic exercise per week, complemented by muscle-strengthening activities on two or more days per week. Before commencing any exercise regimen, particularly if you have an existing liver condition or other medical concerns, it's advisable to consult with your healthcare provider.

LIVER CIRRHOSIS DIET RECIPES

Grilled Salmon with Dill Yogurt Sauce

Ingredients:

- Salmon fillets

- Greek yogurt

- Fresh dill, chopped

- Lemon juice

- Garlic, minced

- Salt and pepper to taste

Instructions:

- Preheat grill to medium-high heat.

- Season salmon fillets with salt, pepper, minced garlic, and lemon juice.

- Grill salmon for 4-5 minutes on each side, or until cooked through.

- In a bowl, mix Greek yogurt with chopped dill and a squeeze of lemon juice.

- Serve grilled salmon with dill yogurt sauce on the side.

Sesame Ginger Tofu Stir-Fry

Ingredients:

- Firm tofu, cubed

- Soy sauce

- Rice vinegar

- Sesame oil

- Fresh ginger, grated

- Garlic, minced

- Mixed vegetables (such as bell peppers, broccoli, and snap peas)

- Cooked brown rice

- Sesame seeds (for garnish)

Instructions:

- In a bowl, whisk together soy sauce, rice vinegar, sesame oil, grated ginger, and minced garlic.

- Marinate cubed tofu in the sauce for 15-20 minutes.

- Heat a skillet over medium-high heat and add marinated tofu.

- Cook until tofu is golden brown on all sides, then remove from the skillet.

- In the same skillet, stir-fry mixed vegetables until tender-crisp.

- Add cooked brown rice and tofu back to the skillet, toss to combine.

- Serve tofu stir-fry garnished with sesame seeds.

Baked Sweet Potato Fries

Ingredients:

- Sweet potatoes, peeled and cut into fries

- Olive oil

- Paprika

- Garlic powder

- Salt and pepper to taste

Instructions:

- Preheat oven to 425°F (220°C) and line a baking sheet with parchment paper.

- In a bowl, toss sweet potato fries with olive oil, paprika, garlic powder, salt, and pepper until evenly coated.

- Arrange fries in a single layer on the prepared baking sheet.

- Bake for 25-30 minutes, flipping halfway through, until fries are crispy and golden brown.

- Serve hot as a healthy side dish.

Mushroom and Spinach Quiche

Ingredients:

- Pie crust (homemade or store-bought)

- Eggs

- Milk or cream

- Mushrooms, sliced

- Fresh spinach, chopped

- Onion, diced

- Garlic, minced

- Olive oil

- Salt and pepper to taste

Instructions:

- Preheat oven to 375°F (190°C).

- In a skillet, heat olive oil over medium heat and sauté diced onion until translucent.

- Add minced garlic, sliced mushrooms, and chopped spinach, cook until mushrooms release their liquid and spinach wilts.

- Season with salt and pepper to taste, then remove from heat.

- In a bowl, whisk together eggs and milk or cream until well combined.

- Roll out pie crust and place it in a pie dish.

- Spread mushroom and spinach mixture evenly over the pie crust.

- Pour egg mixture over the vegetables.

- Bake for 35-40 minutes, or until the quiche is set and golden brown.

- Let cool slightly before slicing and serving.

Zucchini Noodles with Pesto and Cherry Tomatoes

Ingredients:

- Zucchini, spiralized into noodles

- Cherry tomatoes, halved

- Pesto sauce (homemade or store-bought)

- Parmesan cheese, grated (optional)

- Pine nuts, toasted (optional)

Instructions:

- In a skillet, heat a little olive oil over medium heat.

- Add zucchini noodles and cherry tomatoes to the skillet.

- Sauté for 2-3 minutes until zucchini noodles are tender.

- Stir in pesto sauce and toss until everything is well coated.

- Remove from heat and sprinkle with grated Parmesan cheese and toasted pine nuts if desired.

- Serve immediately as a light and flavorful meal.

Turmeric Cauliflower Rice

Ingredients:

- Cauliflower, grated or processed into rice-like texture

- Turmeric powder

- Cumin seeds

- Garlic powder

- Olive oil

- Salt and pepper to taste

Instructions:

- Heat olive oil in a skillet over medium heat.

- Add cumin seeds and sauté for a minute until fragrant.

- Add grated cauliflower to the skillet and stir well.

- Season with turmeric powder, garlic powder, salt, and pepper.

- Cook for 5-7 minutes, stirring occasionally, until cauliflower is tender.

- Serve turmeric cauliflower rice as a nutritious and colorful side dish.

Baked Pears with Honey and Cinnamon
35

Ingredients:

- Pears, halved and cored

- Honey

- Cinnamon

- Walnuts, chopped (optional)

- Greek yogurt (optional)

Instructions:

- Preheat oven to 375°F (190°C).

- Place pear halves, cut side up, on a baking sheet lined with parchment paper.

- Drizzle honey over the pears and sprinkle with cinnamon.

- Bake for 20-25 minutes, or until pears are soft and caramelized.

- Serve baked pears warm, optionally topped with chopped walnuts and a dollop of Greek yogurt.

Salmon and Avocado Salad

Ingredients:

- Fresh salmon fillet

- Mixed salad greens

- Avocado, sliced

- Cherry tomatoes, halved

- Cucumber, sliced

- Red onion, thinly sliced

- Olive oil

- Lemon juice

- Salt and pepper to taste

Instructions:

- Season the salmon fillet with salt and pepper, then grill or bake until cooked through.

- In a large bowl, combine mixed salad greens, sliced avocado, halved cherry tomatoes, sliced cucumber, and thinly sliced red onion.

- Drizzle olive oil and lemon juice over the salad, then toss gently to coat.

- Break the grilled salmon into chunks and add to the salad.

- Serve immediately as a nutritious and satisfying meal.

Quinoa and Vegetable Stir-Fry

Ingredients:

- Quinoa

- Assorted vegetables (such as bell peppers, broccoli, carrots, and snap peas)

- Garlic, minced

- Low-sodium soy sauce

- Olive oil

Instructions:

- Cook quinoa according to package instructions.

- In a large skillet, heat olive oil over medium heat. Add minced garlic and sauté until fragrant.

- Add assorted vegetables to the skillet and stir-fry until tender-crisp.

- Stir in cooked quinoa and soy sauce, tossing until well combined and heated through.

- Serve hot as a nutritious and filling meal.

Turkey and Vegetable Skewers

Ingredients:

- Turkey breast, cut into chunks

- Assorted vegetables (such as cherry tomatoes, zucchini, bell peppers, and mushrooms)

- Olive oil

- Lemon juice

- Italian seasoning

- Salt and pepper to taste

Instructions:

- Preheat grill to medium-high heat.

- Thread turkey chunks and assorted vegetables onto skewers.

- Drizzle olive oil and lemon juice over the skewers, then sprinkle with Italian seasoning, salt, and pepper.

- Grill the skewers for about 8-10 minutes, turning occasionally, until turkey is cooked through and vegetables are tender.

- Serve hot with a side of cooked quinoa or brown rice.

Mango and Avocado Salad with Grilled Chicken

Ingredients:

- Chicken breast

- Ripe mango, diced

- Ripe avocado, diced

- Mixed salad greens

- Red onion, thinly sliced

- Fresh cilantro, chopped

- Lime juice

- Extra virgin olive oil

- Salt and pepper to taste

Instructions:

- Season the chicken breast with salt and pepper, then grill until cooked through.

- In a large bowl, combine diced mango, avocado, mixed salad greens, thinly sliced red onion, and chopped fresh cilantro.

- Drizzle lime juice and extra virgin olive oil over the salad, then season with salt and pepper.

- Slice the grilled chicken breast and arrange on top of the salad.

- Serve immediately as a refreshing and nutritious meal.

Baked Cod with Tomato and Basil

Ingredients:

- Cod fillets

- Fresh tomatoes, sliced

- Fresh basil leaves

- Garlic, minced

- Olive oil

- Lemon juice

- Salt and pepper to taste

Instructions:

- Preheat oven to 375°F (190°C).

- Place cod fillets in a baking dish and season with minced garlic, salt, and pepper.

- Arrange sliced tomatoes and fresh basil leaves on top of the cod fillets.

- Drizzle olive oil and lemon juice over the fish.

- Bake in the preheated oven for about 15-20 minutes, or until fish is cooked through and flakes easily with a fork.

- Serve hot with a side of steamed vegetables or whole grain couscous.

Vegetable Lentil Soup

Ingredients:

- Lentils

- Assorted vegetables (such as carrots, celery, onions, and kale)

- Low-sodium vegetable broth

- Garlic, minced

- Ground cumin

- Paprika

- Olive oil

- Salt and pepper to taste

Instructions:

- Rinse lentils under cold water and drain.

- In a large pot, heat olive oil over medium heat. Add minced garlic and sauté until fragrant.

- Add assorted vegetables to the pot and cook until softened.

- Stir in lentils, ground cumin, paprika, and low-sodium vegetable broth.

- Bring the soup to a boil, then reduce heat and simmer for about 25-30 minutes, or until lentils are tender.

- Season with salt and pepper to taste before serving hot.

Asian-Inspired Baked Tofu

Ingredients:

- Firm tofu, sliced into cubes or rectangles

- Soy sauce

- Rice vinegar

- Sesame oil

- Ginger, grated

- Garlic, minced

- Green onions, chopped (for garnish)

Instructions:

- Preheat oven to 375°F (190°C) and line a baking sheet with parchment paper.

- In a bowl, whisk together soy sauce, rice vinegar, sesame oil, grated ginger, and minced garlic.

- Marinate tofu cubes in the sauce for at least 30 minutes.

- Arrange marinated tofu on the prepared baking sheet.

- Bake for 25-30 minutes, flipping halfway through, until tofu is golden brown and crispy.

- Garnish with chopped green onions before serving.

Beet and Carrot Salad with Citrus Dressing

Ingredients:

- Beets, cooked and sliced

- Carrots, grated

- Oranges, segmented

- Lemon juice

- Olive oil

- Honey

- Dijon mustard

- Fresh parsley, chopped

- Salt and pepper to taste

Instructions:

- In a bowl, whisk together lemon juice, olive oil, honey, Dijon mustard, salt, and pepper to make the dressing.

- Arrange cooked and sliced beets, grated carrots, and segmented oranges on a serving platter.

- Drizzle the citrus dressing over the salad.

- Garnish with chopped fresh parsley before serving.

Sardine and White Bean Salad

Ingredients:

- Canned sardines in olive oil

- Cannellini beans, drained and rinsed

- Cherry tomatoes, halved

- Red onion, thinly sliced

- Fresh basil leaves, torn

- Red wine vinegar

- Extra virgin olive oil

- Salt and pepper to taste

Instructions:

- In a large bowl, combine canned sardines (with oil), cannellini beans, halved cherry tomatoes, thinly sliced red onion, and torn fresh basil leaves.

- Drizzle with red wine vinegar and extra virgin olive oil.

- Season with salt and pepper to taste.

- Toss gently to combine.

- Serve chilled or at room temperature.

Tofu and Vegetable Curry

Ingredients:

- Firm tofu, cubed

- Mixed vegetables (such as bell peppers, broccoli, and cauliflower)

- Coconut milk

- Red curry paste

- Onion, chopped

- Garlic, minced

- Ginger, grated

- Vegetable broth

- Soy sauce

- Olive oil

- Fresh cilantro, chopped (for garnish)

Instructions:

55

- In a large skillet or wok, heat olive oil over medium heat.

- Add chopped onion, minced garlic, and grated ginger. Sauté until fragrant.

- Stir in red curry paste and cook for a minute.

- Add cubed tofu and mixed vegetables. Cook until vegetables are tender-crisp.

- Pour in coconut milk and vegetable broth. Bring to a simmer.

- Season with soy sauce to taste.

- Simmer for a few minutes until the flavors meld together.

- Garnish with chopped fresh cilantro before serving.

Stuffed Bell Peppers with Quinoa and Lentils

Ingredients:

- Bell peppers

- Quinoa, cooked

- Lentils, cooked

- Onion, chopped

- Garlic, minced

- Tomato sauce

- Italian seasoning

- Salt and pepper to taste

- Shredded mozzarella cheese (optional)

Instructions:

- Preheat oven to 375°F (190°C).

- Cut the tops off bell peppers and remove seeds and membranes.

- In a skillet, sauté chopped onion and minced garlic until softened.

- Stir in cooked quinoa, cooked lentils, tomato sauce, Italian seasoning, salt, and pepper.

- Stuff bell peppers with the quinoa and lentil mixture.

- Place stuffed bell peppers in a baking dish. If desired, sprinkle shredded mozzarella cheese on top.

- Cover with foil and bake for 25-30 minutes.

- Remove foil and bake for an additional 10 minutes, or until peppers are tender and cheese is melted and bubbly.

Zucchini and Tomato Gratin

Ingredients:

- Zucchini, thinly sliced

- Tomatoes, thinly sliced

- Onion, thinly sliced

- Garlic, minced

- Fresh thyme leaves

- Parmesan cheese, grated

- Olive oil

- Salt and pepper to taste

Instructions:

- Preheat oven to 375°F (190°C).

- In a skillet, heat olive oil over medium heat. Add minced garlic and thinly sliced onion. Sauté until softened.

- Layer thinly sliced zucchini and tomatoes in a baking dish, alternating between the two.

- Sprinkle sautéed onion and garlic over the zucchini and tomatoes.

- Season with fresh thyme leaves, salt, and pepper.

- Sprinkle grated Parmesan cheese on top.

- Cover with foil and bake for 25-30 minutes.

- Remove foil and bake for an additional 10 minutes, or until vegetables are tender and cheese is golden brown.

Saffron-infused Chicken and Barley Soup

Ingredients:

- Chicken thighs, boneless and skinless

- Barley

- Carrots, diced

- Celery, diced

- Onion, chopped

- Garlic, minced

- Saffron threads

- Chicken broth

- Olive oil

- Fresh parsley, chopped

- Salt and pepper to taste

Instructions:

- In a large pot, heat olive oil over medium heat.

- Add chopped onion, minced garlic, diced carrots, and diced celery. Sauté until softened.

- Add boneless chicken thighs and cook until lightly browned.

- Pour in chicken broth and bring to a simmer.

- Stir in barley and saffron threads.

- Simmer for about 30-40 minutes, or until barley is tender and chicken is cooked through.

- Season with salt and pepper to taste.

- Garnish with chopped fresh parsley before serving.

Miso Glazed Eggplant with Quinoa

Ingredients:

- Eggplant, sliced into rounds

- Quinoa

- White miso paste

- Soy sauce

- Rice vinegar

- Mirin

- Brown sugar

- Garlic, minced

- Sesame seeds (for garnish)

Instructions:

- Cook quinoa according to package instructions.

- In a bowl, whisk together white miso paste, soy sauce, rice vinegar, mirin, brown sugar, and minced garlic to make the glaze.

- Brush both sides of eggplant slices with the miso glaze.

- Grill or broil the eggplant slices until tender and caramelized.

- Serve the grilled miso eggplant over cooked quinoa.

- Garnish with sesame seeds before serving.

Baked Stuffed Acorn Squash with Wild Rice and Cranberries

Ingredients:

- Acorn squash, halved and seeds removed

- Wild rice

- Dried cranberries

- Pecans, chopped

- Maple syrup

- Cinnamon

- Nutmeg

- Olive oil

- Salt and pepper to taste

Instructions:

- Preheat oven to 375°F (190°C).

- Rub acorn squash halves with olive oil and season with salt and pepper.

- Place squash halves cut-side down on a baking sheet and roast for 25-30 minutes, or until tender.

- In the meantime, cook wild rice according to package instructions.

- In a bowl, mix cooked wild rice with dried cranberries, chopped pecans, maple syrup, cinnamon, and nutmeg.

- Stuff the roasted acorn squash halves with the wild rice mixture.

- Return stuffed squash to the oven and bake for another 15-20 minutes.

- Serve hot as a hearty and nutritious meal.

Spaghetti Squash Pad Thai

Ingredients:

- Spaghetti squash

- Shrimp, peeled and deveined

- Bean sprouts

- Scallions, sliced

- Red bell pepper, thinly sliced

- Carrot, julienned

- Garlic, minced

- Eggs, beaten

- Peanuts, chopped (for garnish)

- Fresh cilantro, chopped (for garnish)

- Lime wedges (for serving)

- Pad Thai sauce (store-bought or homemade)

Instructions:

- Preheat oven to 375°F (190°C).

- Cut spaghetti squash in half lengthwise and remove seeds.

- Place squash halves cut-side down on a baking sheet lined with parchment paper.

- Bake for 40-50 minutes, or until squash is tender and easily pierced with a fork.

- In a skillet, heat olive oil over medium heat.

- Add minced garlic, sliced red bell pepper, and julienned carrot. Sauté until vegetables are tender.

- Push vegetables to one side of the skillet and pour beaten eggs into the other side. Scramble until cooked.

- Add shrimp to the skillet and cook until pink and opaque.

- Scrape the cooked spaghetti squash into the skillet using a fork.

- Pour Pad Thai sauce over the mixture and toss until well combined.

- Stir in bean sprouts and sliced scallions.

- Garnish with chopped peanuts and fresh cilantro.

- Serve hot with lime wedges on the side.

Grilled Halibut with Mango Salsa

Ingredients:

- Halibut fillets

- Mango, diced

- Red bell pepper, diced

- Red onion, finely chopped

- Cilantro, chopped

- Lime juice

- Olive oil

- Salt and pepper to taste

Instructions:

- Preheat grill to medium-high heat.

- Season halibut fillets with olive oil, salt, and pepper.

- Grill halibut for 4-5 minutes per side, or until cooked through.

- In a bowl, combine diced mango, red bell pepper, red onion, cilantro, lime juice, olive oil, salt, and pepper to make the salsa.

- Serve grilled halibut topped with mango salsa.

Stuffed Portobello Mushrooms with Quinoa and Spinach

Ingredients:

- Portobello mushrooms

- Quinoa, cooked

- Spinach, chopped

- Garlic, minced

- Red bell pepper, diced

- Feta cheese, crumbled

- Olive oil

- Balsamic vinegar

- Salt and pepper to taste

Instructions:

- Preheat oven to 375°F (190°C).

- Remove stems from portobello mushrooms and scoop out

  the gills.

- In a skillet, heat olive oil over medium heat. Add minced garlic and diced red bell pepper, sauté until softened.

- Stir in chopped spinach and cooked quinoa, cook until spinach wilts.

- Season with salt and pepper to taste.

- Fill portobello mushrooms with the quinoa and spinach mixture.

- Place stuffed mushrooms on a baking sheet and bake for 20-25 minutes.

- Drizzle with balsamic vinegar before serving.

Cucumber and Avocado Gazpacho

Ingredients:

- Cucumbers, peeled and chopped

- Avocado, peeled and diced

- Green onions, chopped

- Jalapeño pepper, seeded and chopped

- Garlic, minced

- Lime juice

- Greek yogurt

- Fresh cilantro, chopped

- Salt and pepper to taste

Instructions:

- In a blender, combine chopped cucumbers, diced avocado, chopped green onions, chopped jalapeño pepper, minced garlic, lime juice, Greek yogurt, fresh cilantro, salt, and pepper.

- Blend until smooth and creamy.

- Chill in the refrigerator for at least 1 hour before serving.

- Garnish with additional chopped cilantro before serving.

Cauliflower Rice Sushi Rolls

Ingredients:

- Cauliflower, grated or processed into rice-like texture

- Nori seaweed sheets

- Avocado, thinly sliced

- Cucumber, thinly sliced

- Carrot, thinly sliced

- Cooked crab or shrimp (optional)

- Rice vinegar

- Soy sauce (reduced-sodium)

- Wasabi and pickled ginger (optional, for serving)

Instructions:

- Prepare cauliflower rice by grating or processing cauliflower florets.

- Season cauliflower rice with a splash of rice vinegar.

- Place a nori seaweed sheet on a sushi rolling mat or clean kitchen towel.

- Spread a thin layer of cauliflower rice over the nori sheet.

- Arrange avocado slices, cucumber, carrot, and cooked crab or shrimp (if using) along the center of the rice.

- Carefully roll the nori sheet tightly around the fillings using the sushi rolling mat or towel.

- Slice the sushi roll into bite-sized pieces using a sharp knife.

- Serve with reduced-sodium soy sauce, wasabi, and pickled ginger.

Quinoa Stuffed Bell Peppers with Turkey

Ingredients:

- Bell peppers
- Quinoa, cooked
- Lean ground turkey
- Onion, diced
- Garlic, minced
- Tomato sauce (unsweetened)
- Italian seasoning
- Olive oil
- Salt and pepper to taste

Instructions:

- Preheat oven to 375°F (190°C).
- Cut the tops off bell peppers and remove seeds.
- In a skillet, heat olive oil over medium heat.

- Sauté diced onion and minced garlic until softened.

- Add ground turkey to the skillet and cook until browned.

- Stir in cooked quinoa, tomato sauce, and Italian seasoning. Cook until heated through.

- Season with salt and pepper to taste.

- Stuff bell peppers with the quinoa and turkey mixture.

- Place stuffed peppers in a baking dish and cover with foil.

- Bake for 25-30 minutes, then remove foil and bake for an additional 10 minutes.

Baked Garlic Herb Tofu

Ingredients:

- Firm tofu, sliced into rectangles

- Olive oil

- Garlic powder

- Dried basil

- Dried oregano

- Salt and pepper to taste

Instructions:

- Preheat oven to 375°F (190°C).

- Place tofu slices on a baking sheet lined with parchment paper.

- Drizzle tofu with olive oil and sprinkle with garlic powder, dried basil, dried oregano, salt, and pepper.

- Bake for 25-30 minutes, or until tofu is golden brown and crispy on the edges.

- Serve as a protein-rich side dish or add to salads and stir-

  fries.

Miso Glazed Salmon

Ingredients:

- Salmon fillets

- White miso paste

- Soy sauce (reduced-sodium)

- Mirin

- Honey or maple syrup

- Rice vinegar

- Sesame oil

- Fresh ginger, grated

- Garlic, minced

Instructions:

- In a bowl, whisk together white miso paste, reduced-sodium soy sauce, mirin, honey or maple syrup, rice vinegar, sesame oil, grated ginger, and minced garlic to make the glaze.

- Place salmon fillets on a baking sheet lined with parchment paper.

- Brush salmon fillets with the miso glaze.

- Bake in a preheated oven at 400°F (200°C) for 12-15 minutes, or until salmon is cooked through and flakes easily with a fork.

- Serve hot with steamed vegetables or brown rice.

THANKS FOR

READING

THIS BOOK.